Copycat Re[c]...

Begin...

Easy Step-by-Step Recipe Cookbook with Exclusive Tips and Tricks.

Enjoy the best Dishes from Texas Roadhouse, Chipotle, Cheesecake Factory, Cracker Barrel and Panera.

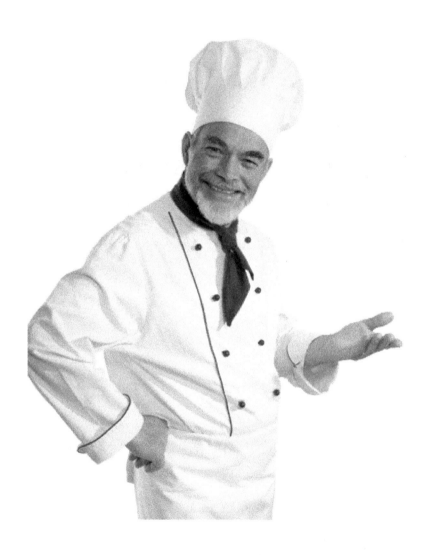

TABLE OF CONTENTS

INTRODUCTION

Thank you for purchasing this book.

Copycat recipes might taste almost like recipes from eateries. Many restaurant recipes are completed with every ingredient that anybody can discover in their kitchen. By recreating the recipe reception, you'll replicate several of your favorite restaurant meals. Some restaurant recipes aren't really special or made with secret ingredients, many of the restaurant's hottest dishes are really classic dishes we already know and love. You will find step-by-step instructions for all those amazing dishes that attract people to restaurants, and you will be sure the food has been cooked under hygienic conditions as you are going to form it yourself. To cook those meals, you do not need to be a master chef. All the recipes during this book use key ingredients available in any grocery. No got to buy fancy equipment, because the cooking techniques are simple. Making use of this book

You can find recommendations on the way to achieve restaurant-feeling reception. You'll get an inventory of basic cookware and appliances in your kitchen also as the way to store your pantry to organize some wonderful dishes. Recipes are organized into chapters based on the typical ingredients for each category. For instance, the seafood chapter includes recipes for shrimp, crab cakes, oysters and salmon while the poultry chapter includes recipes for chicken and duck.

This guide is going to be offered on the way to select the simplest and freshest ingredients. The essential cooking language and methods utilized in this book also will be learned. Many key considerations that require to be addressed when building a restaurant experience reception are fixing an attractive table and displaying the food within the most Appealing way.

You'll use certain recipes and make your own replacements for a meal freed from calories or sugar. Since you already know what the dish will taste like beforehand, you recognize you'll enjoy it before you begin cooking.

Portion management may be a major issue in today's restaurant industry. Every meal on an enormous plate is served with the thought that more are going to be better. Majority of diet books commend you eat just half the serving of an entrée when eating out and put the rest during a box to travel.

Cooking in your restaurant style reception is not difficult. You will get step-by-step directions for numerous recipes that you could make inside the comfort and ease of your own home. A number of the recipes inside this book are just as good as those found in expensive restaurants.

Cooking reception means you can control what percentage calories you eat. You'll also take an opportunity from the meal and a couple of hours later have cake and occasional, which are some things you would not neutralize a restaurant. Cloning recipes are often a pleasant activity during which the entire family will participate. in only a sitting, you'll be skilled of fixing plates from several diverse restaurants. I hope that this book will make you want to cook. Enjoy it and have fun!

SALAD RECIPES

Popeye's Caesar Low Carb Dressing Salad

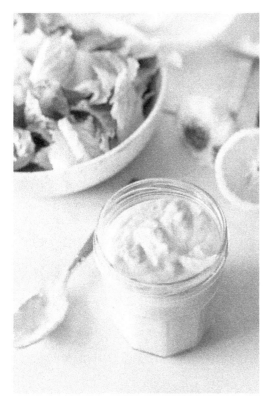

Preparation Time: 16 minutes

Cooking Time: 13 minutes

Servings: 3

Ingredients

- 2 chickens
- Dijon Mustard 1 tbsp
- 1 crushed garlic clove
- 3 Anchovies
- 1 tsp of White Pepper
- 2-3 pinches of salt
- 17 fl. oz. of medium flavored olive oil
- 2 oz grated Parmesan cheese
- 1/3 cup of finely chopped Parsley
- Lemon Juice 3 tbsp

Direction

1. In a food processor, place the eggs, mustard, garlic, anchovies, salt, and pepper and combine at medium / high speed for 3 minutes or until well blended.
2. Drop the velocity well below medium and very slowly, in a thin stream, apply the oil. It will allow the dressing to break if the oil is used too soon.
3. Attach the parmesan cheese, sliced parsley, and lemon juice and mix until mixed.
4. If needed, taste and change the seasoning. To thin it, apply 2-3 teaspoons of warm water if the dressing is too thick.

5. Serve it drizzled, or use it as a dipping sauce, over your favorite salad.

Nutrition 21 Calories 1g Protein 1g Fat

Subway's Frittata Keto with New Spinach

Preparation Time: 9 minutes

Cooking Time: 16 minutes

Servings: 4

Ingredients

- 5 oz. Bacon or chorizo sliced
- 2 tbsp of butter
- 8 oz. New spinach
- 8 eggs
- 1 cup of healthy ice cream
- 5 oz. Cheese shredded
- Salt and pepper

Direction

1. Oven preheat to 175 ° C (350 ° F). Oven. Grate a ramekin alone or a pan with a 9x9 baker.
2. Freeze the bacon in the butter until soft, medium heat. Then whisk and wilt the spinach. Get the pot off the heat and set it aside.
3. Whisk eggs and milk together and dump them into a bakery or ramekin.

4. Using it in the middle of the oven to add the bacon, spinach and cheese. Bake until fair and golden brown on top for around 25-30 minutes.

Nutrition 661 Calories 59g Fat 27g Protein

Hardee's & Carl's Jr.'s Sundried Asparagus and Roasted Tomatoes Pasta

Preparation Time: 11 minutes

Cooking Time: 19 minutes

Servings: 5

Ingredients

- Medium-sized spaghetti 8 ounces.
- Trimmed 1 pound of asparagus.
- 2 olive oil cu charts.
- 1/2 cup of pesto basil.
- 1/3 cup of sun-dried tomatoes drained in olive oil
- Mozzarella cubes 1/3 cup sliced
- Egg fried, to be eaten

Direction

1. Preheat oven to 425 F. Preheat oven. Baked or coated with nonstick spray lightly oil. Lightly oil.
2. Cook pasta according to label instructions in a big pot of boiling salted water; rinse well.
3. Place the spray in one layer on the prepared bakery mat. Dry the olive oil, salt and pepper to taste; kindly mix. Situate in the oven and roast

for 8-12 minutes, or until soft but crisp. Only let it cool before you break it into 1-inch pieces.

4. In a wide dish mix pasta, asparagus, pesto, sun-dried tomatoes and mozzarella.

5. Serve with a fried egg as soon as required.

Nutrition 457 calories 17g protein 15g fat

Jack in the Box's Salad Steak Fajita

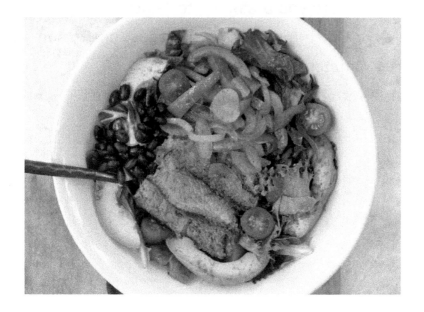

Preparation Time: 9 minutes

Cooking Time: 13 minutes

Servings: 4

Ingredients

- 2 olive oil teaspoons, cut.
- 1 ointment, slim cut
- Slimly cut 1 red bell pepper
- 1 orange pepper thinly sliced
- 1 bell of green pepper, fine cut
- 8 Roman cups of salad hacked
- 1 avocado, cut in half, seeded, scratched and sliced finely

For cilantro chalk dressing

- 1 cup of loose, trimmed coriander.
- 1/2 cup of milk with whips.
- 2 mayonnaise ounces
- 2 cloves of garlic.
- 1 lime savory
- Pinch of salt
- Olive oil 1/4 cup
- 2 apple cider teaspoons of vinegar

Due to the steak

- Olive Oil 1/4 cup
- 2 garlic cloves, hairy
- 1 lime savory
- 1 cumin soil tea cu char.
- 1 teaspoon of chili powder
- 1 teaspoon of preserved oregano
- 1/2 onion tea powder
- Black pepper and casher salt freshly roasted
- Flank steak 2 kg

Direction

1. In food processor bowls to make cilantro lime dressing, mix coriander, savory sauce, mayonnaise, ginger, lime juice and salt. In a slow stream apply the olive oil and vinegar to the engine; set aside.

2. Stir olive oil, garlic, lime juice, cumin, chili powder, oregano and onion pulp together in a small cup; season with salt and pepper to taste.

3. In a gallon bag or large tub, mix steak and marinade; marinate, turning, rotate occasionally, for at least 30 minutes. Drain and cut the steak from the marinade.

4. Fire a medium-high heat one tablespoon of olive oil in a barbecue dish. Work in a lot, cook the steak and toss once, at the optimum temperature, around 3-4 minutes per hand, average rare. Pull away from the heat and rest 10 minutes before slicing the grain thinly.

5. Stir in the skillet, applying the onion and roast, until the onion is translucent and gently caramelized, for about 7-8 minutes; leave aside.

6. Cook 1 tablespoon of olive oil in the skillet. Connect the bell peppers and boil until soft and mildly caramelized for around 8-10 minutes, stirring often; set aside.

7. Into a bowl, put the Roman salad in a large bowl; cover with tomato, pep, steak, and avocado arranged lines.

8. Serve as soon as possible with coriander dressing.

Nutrition 699 calories 50g protein 42g fat

Chipotle's Burrito Easy Bowles

Preparation Time: 9 minutes

Cooking Time: 12 minutes

Servings: 4

Ingredients

- Uncooked 1 cup of rice
- 1 cup of salsa, whether homemade or shopping.
- Three cups hairy Roman lettuce
- 1 can be kernel whole maize (15.25 ounce), drained maize,
- 1 black, drained and rinsed (15-ounce) beans
- Two Roma tomatoes, diced
- 1 avocado, stemmed, peeled and sliced. 1 avocado
- 2 fresh coriander leaves teaspoons
- With the chipotle cream sauce
- 1 sample of milk whipped
- 1 tablespoon paste *
- 1 pinched garlic clove
- 1 lime savory
- Taste 1/4 teaspoon of salt or more

Direction

1. To produce a chipotle cream sauce, whisk in sour cream, chipotle paste, garlic, lime juice and salt.
2. Cook the rice in a wide saucepan of 1 1/2 cups of water according to packaging directions and keep it cold and whisk in a salsa.
3. Divide the meal into serving dishes, then top with broccoli, maize, black beans, onions, avocados then cilantro.
4. Serve fast, chipotle milk drizzled in sauce.

Nutrition 638 calories 26g protein 39g fat

Smoothie King's Valle in Fruit Quinoa

Preparation Time: 9 minutes

Cooking Time: 12 minutes

Servings: 3

Ingredients

- 2 tables of cooked quinoa
- 1 stick, skinned and cut
- Divide in quarters 1 cup of strawberries.
- 1/2 cup of fatty fruit
- 2 pine nuts cups 2
- Hammered mint leaves for garnish
- The Lemon's Vinaigrette
- Olive Oil 1/4 cup
- Apple cider 1/4 cup vinegar
- 1 lemon zest
- 3 tablespoons of fried citrus juice
- 1 sugar tablespoon

Direction

1. In a small cup, whisk the olive oil, the cider vinegar, the citrus fruit and the juice with the sugar to make a vinaigrette; reserve.

2. Combine a large dish of quinoa, an apple, strawberries, blueberries and pine nuts. Drop a lemon vinaigrette.

3. Serve promptly, garnished with mint leaves.

Nutrition 799 calories 40g protein 36g fat

Applebee's Kohlslaw Keto

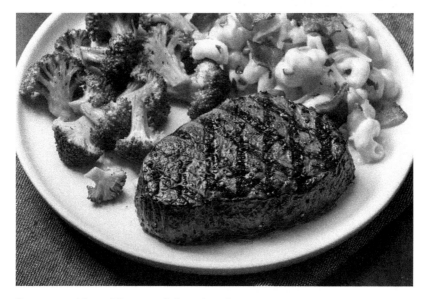

Preparation Time: 11 minutes

Cooking Time: 8 minutes

Servings: 4

Ingredients

- 1 pound of kohlrabies
- 1 cup of mayonnaise or vegan mayonnaise
- Salt and potato
- New parsley (optional)

Direction

1. Strip the kohlrabi. Make sure that all rough, woody bits are cut off. Finely shave, slice, and shred it and put it in a tub.

2. Add the mayonnaise and optional fresh herbs. To taste, add salt and pepper.

Nutrition 442 calories 46g protein 25g fat

Starbucks's Coleslaw with Mixed Cabbage

Preparation Time: 12 minutes

Cooking Time: 0 minutes

Servings: 4

Ingredients

- Green cabbage 8 oz.
- 4 ounces of red cabbage
- 4 ounces of kale
- 1 mayonnaise cup
- 1/2 tsp of salt
- 1/2 TL of black pepper field

Direction

1. With a strong knife, mandolin slicer, or a food processor, split the cabbage.
2. Place the mayonnaise, salt, and pepper in a bowl and add them. Stir well and leave to rest for ten minutes.

Nutrition 632 calories 9.2g protein 51g fat

Au Bon Pain's Bacon Cups from Cobb Salad

Preparation Time: 14 minutes

Cooking Time: 16 minutes

Servings: 6

Ingredients

- 12 slices of thin bacon sliced
- 1 cup of thinly sliced romaine lettuce
- 1/2 cup of roasted chicken chopped
- 1/2 chopped California Avocado
- 1 finely cut hardboiled egg
- 1/4 cup of diced tomato
- 2 tbsp optional crumbled blue cheese
- Dressing of preference

Direction

1. To 425F, preheat the oven. Turn a muffin box of the average size upside down and cover with foil, forming the cups nearby.
2. Break 6 of the slices of bacon in half. Fill the bottom of each muffin cup with two halves of bacon in an X pattern. Wind a full-length strip of bacon across each cup's edges so that they are sealed with a toothpick.

3. Bake the cups of bacon to your taste until finished. For crispy bacon, I considered this to be around 35 minutes. Remove to cool for 20 minutes, remove the toothpicks to remove the foil from the cups, and turn them right side up.
4. Divide the cups with the salad, chicken, avocado, egg, tomato, and blue cheese.
5. Top-up and serve with your preferred sauce. Or don't dress at all; without it, they're tasty!

Nutrition 145 Calories 9.9g Fat9.5g Protein

Houlihan's Deviled Eggs Bacon-Avocado Caesar

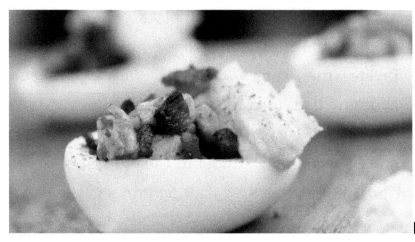

Preparation Time: 1 minutes

Cooking Time: 0 minutes

Servings: 4

Ingredients

- Eggs
- 2 chickens
- 1 tablespoon mayonnaise
- 1/4 teaspoon of mustard Dijon
- 1/8 lemon squeezed
- 1/4 of garlic powder teaspoon (optional; omit if you are allergic to garlic).
- 1/8 teaspoon of pink Himalayan salt
- 1/8 teaspoon of paprika smoked

Filling with Bacon-Avocado

- 1/4 of avocado
- 1 slice of bacon from pasture

Direction

Filling:

1. Chop a 1/4-inch slice of bacon and avocado.
2. In a medium-hot pan, add bacon and cook for 3 minutes or until browned.
3. Attach the avocado and cook for another 3 minutes, then reduce the heat to normal.

Eggs:

1. Carry two quarts to a boil with water. Lower the heat, add the eggs and cook for 8 minutes.
2. For 3 minutes, put the cooked eggs in ice water and then peel and split in half, lengthwise.
3. Remove the yolk from the cut eggs gently and apply the mayonnaise, mustard, lemon, garlic powder, and salt to a food processor and run the processor until the mixture is smooth.
4. Gently spoon the egg white with the bacon-avocado filling. Cover with Caesar egg yolk mixture and sprinkle with smoking paprika, using a spoon, piping bag, or resealable plastic bag with a snipped corner.

Nutrition: 422 Calories 16g Protein 30g Fat

MAIN RECIPES

Lobster-Stuffed Avocado

Preparation Time: 15 minutes

Cooking Time: 5 minutes

Serving: 4

Ingredients:

- 1 tbsp avocado oil mayonnaise
- 1 tbsp lemon juice (fresh)
- 2 tbsp butter (melted)
- 2 cups lobster meat (chopped, cooled at room temperature)
- 2 California avocados (halved, pitted)
- 1 celery stalk (chopped)
- 1 green onion (chopped)
- black pepper
- chives (fresh, chopped)
- salt

Directions:

1. In a bowl, combine the lobster meat, green onion, and celery. Add the mayonnaise, lemon

juice, and butter, then toss lightly to coat evenly. Season with salt and pepper.

2. Use a spoon to scoop out some of the avocado flesh. Just leave about half an inch of flesh Spoon the lobster mixture into the avocado halves—about half a cup for each. Garnish with chives and serve immediately.

Nutrition: 111 Calories 21g Fat 82g Protein

Fried Soft-Shell Crab

Preparation Time: 16 minutes

Cooking Time: 5 minutes

Serving: 2

Ingredients:

- 4 tbsp barbecue sauce
- ½ cup lard
- ½ cup parmesan cheese (powdered)
- 2 eggs (beaten)
- 8 soft shell crabs

Directions:

1. Heat a skillet with lard over medium-high heat. Use a paper towel to pat the crabs dry. Prepare the parmesan and eggs by placing them in separate shallow dishes.
2. Dip one crab into the egg, tap off any excess, and dip into the parmesan cheese. Make sure the crab is coated well and evenly. Drop batches of crabs into the oil and cook for about 2 minutes on each side.
3. Serve the crabs hot with barbecue sauce for dipping.

Nutrition: 121 Calories 23g Fat 83g Protein

Turkey and Stuffing

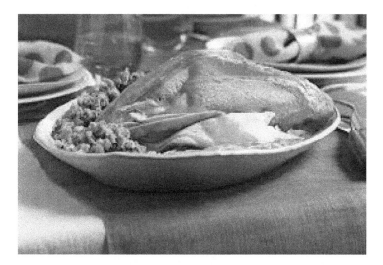

Preparation Time: 10 minutes

Cooking time: 60 minutes

Servings: 4

Ingredients:

- 4 cups day-old cornbread
- 2 cups day-old biscuits
- 1/3 cup chopped onion
- 1 cup diced celery
- 2 tablespoons dried parsley flakes
- 1 teaspoon poultry seasoning
- 1 teaspoon ground sage
- ½ teaspoon coarse ground pepper
- ¼ cup butter or margarine, melted
- 24 ounces chicken broth

- Cooking spray for greasing
- 8 cooked thick turkey breast slices
- 1 cup cranberry sauce
- Favorite sides such as green beans and mashed potatoes

Gravy

- 3 tablespoons butter
- ½ cup diced onions
- 2 tablespoons all-purpose flour
- ¼ teaspoon salt
- ¼ teaspoon pepper
- 1/8 teaspoon dry sage flakes
- 1/8 teaspoon dry parsley flakes
- 1¼ cups milk

Directions:

1. Preheat oven to 400F and spray an 8x8-inch baking dish with cooking spray.
2. In a food processor, add the cornbread and the biscuits. Process until you get a coarse consistency. Alternatively, grate the cornbread and biscuits with a large hole hand grater.
3. In a large bowl, stir together the onion, celery, grated cornbread and biscuits, parsley, poultry seasoning, sage, and pepper.

4. Add the butter and chicken broth to the dry stuffing and mix to combine well.

5. Spread the stuffing evenly to the prepared baking dish. Bake uncovered for 1 hour or until golden brown.

6. Warm-up the turkey in foil in the oven for 15-20 minutes or until warmed through.

7. Prepare the gravy by whisking the dry gravy ingredients together in a bowl. Cook butter in a saucepan at medium heat and add the onions. Stir fry over medium-low heat until fragrant and tender. Add the dry ingredients. Whisk continuously, stirring thoroughly to remove lumps. When the flour begins to brown, slowly whisk in the milk. Continue cooking and whisking for about 2-3 minutes or until the mixture thickens.

8. To serve, add two slices of turkey to each plate and top with some gravy. Add some stuffing, top with some more of the gravy. Add some cranberry sauce and favorite sides.

Nutrition: 123 Calories 22g Fat 80g Protein

Clam Chowder

Preparation Time: 5 minutes

Cooking Time: 6 hours

Servings: 6

Ingredients:

- 20-ounce wild-caught baby clams, with juice
- ½ cup chopped scallion
- ½ cup chopped celery
- 1 teaspoon salt
- 1 teaspoon ground black pepper
- 1 teaspoon dried thyme
- 1 tablespoon avocado oil
- 2 cups coconut cream, full-fat
- 2 cups chicken broth

Directions:

1. Grease a 6-quart slow cooker with oil, then add ingredients and stir until mixed. Plug in the slow cooker, shut with lid and cook for 4 to 6 hours at low heat setting or until cooked through. Serve straightaway.

Nutrition: 112 Calories 21g Fat 79g Protein

Poached Salmon

Preparation Time: 5 minutes

Cooking Time: 3 hours and 35 minutes

Servings: 4

Ingredients:

- 4 steaks of wild-caught salmon
- 1 medium white onion, peeled and sliced
- 2 teaspoons minced garlic
- 1/2 teaspoon salt
- 1/8 teaspoon ground white pepper
- 1/2 teaspoon dried dill weed
- 2 tablespoons avocado oil
- 2 tablespoons unsalted butter
- 2 tablespoons lemon juice

1 cup water

Directions:

2. Place butter in a 4-quart slow cooker, then add salmon and drizzle with oil. Place remaining ingredients in a medium saucepan, stir until mixed and bring the mixture to boil over high heat.

3. Then pour this mixture all over salmon and shut with lid. Plug in the slow cooker and cook salmon for 3 hours and 30 minutes at low heat

setting or until salmon is tender. Serve straightaway.

Nutrition: 113 Calories 23g Fat 78g Protein

The Mexican Pizza

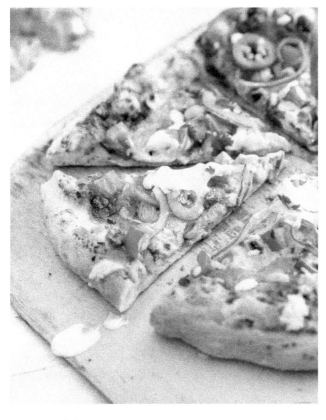

Preparation

Time: 30 minutes

Cooking Time: 12 minutes

Servings: 4

Ingredients:

- ½ pound ground beef
- ½ teaspoon salt
- ¼ teaspoon onion, finely chopped
- ¼ teaspoon paprika
- 1½ teaspoon chili powder

- 2 tablespoons water
- 1 cup vegetable oil
- 8 6-inch flour tortillas
- 1 16-ounce can re-fried beans
- 2/3 cup picante sauce
- 1/3 cup tomato, finely chopped
- 1 cup cheddar cheese, grated
- 1 cup Colby jack cheese, grated
- ¼ cup green onion, diced
- ¼ cup black olives, chopped

Directions:

1. Preheat oven to 400°F.
2. In a skillet, sauté beef on medium heat. Once brown, drain. Then stir in salt, onions, paprika, chili powder, and water. While continuously stirring, cook for an additional 10 minutes.
3. In a separate skillet add oil and heat over medium-high. Cook tortilla for about 30 seconds on both sides or until golden brown. Use a fork to pierce any bubbles forming on the tortillas. Transfer onto a plate lined with paper towels.
4. Microwave refried beans on high for about 30 seconds or until warm.
5. To build each pizza, coat 1/3 cup beans on tortilla followed by 1/3 cup cooked beef. Top

with a second tortilla. Cover with 2 tablespoons picante sauce, then equal amounts of tomatoes, cheeses, green onions, and olives. This makes a total of 4 pizzas.

6. Place prepared pizzas on baking sheet. Bake for 9 minutes. Serve.

Nutrition: 218 Calories 90g Fat 39g Protein

Olive Garden's Chicken Margherita

Preparation Time: 30 min

Cooking Time: 30 minutes

Servings: 4

Ingredients:

- Whole-wheat spaghetti (8 oz. uncooked)
- Chicken breast halves (4 @ 5 oz. each skinless & boneless)
- Pepper (.5 tsp.)
- Bruschetta topping (1 cup prepared)
- Shredded Italian cheese blend (.33 cup)
- Grated parmesan cheese (2 tbsp.)

Directions:

1. Warm the oven broiler. Prepare the spaghetti according to the package instructions and drain in a colander.
2. Use a meat mallet to pound the chicken into a 1/2-inch thickness. Sprinkle each piece using pepper.
3. Spritz a skillet with cooking oil spray. Cook the chicken using the medium temperature setting for five to six minutes per side.
4. Transfer the meat to an eight-inch square baking pan. Scoop a portion of the bruschetta

topping over the chicken and garnish with the cheeses.

5. Broil it about three to four inches from the burner elements (5-6 min.) or until the cheese is golden brown. Serve with the spaghetti.

Note: Look for the bruschetta topping in your grocer's deli case or the pasta aisle.

Nutrition: Calories: 431 Protein: 40 grams Fat: 10 grams Sat. Fats: 4 grams Carbohydrates: 47 grams Sugars: 4 grams Fiber: 8 grams

Olive Garden's Shrimp Fettuccine Alfredo

Preparation Time: 24 min

Cooking Time: 30 minutes

Servings: 5

Ingredients:

- Uncooked fettuccine (12 oz.)
- Olive oil divided (2 tbsp.)
- Jumbo shrimp (1 lb. Uncooked)
- Minced garlic (6 cloves)
- Evaporated milk (12 oz. can)
- Grated parmesan cheese (.25 cup)
- Salt (.5 tsp.)
- Sour cream (.25 cup)
- Drained crabmeat (.5 lb.)
- Fresh basil (.25 cup)

Directions:

1. Prepare the fettuccine according to package instructions, and set it to the side for now.
2. Peel and devein the shrimp.
3. Warm one tablespoon of oil in a skillet using the med-high temperature setting.

4. Add the shrimp and simmer until they have turned pink (4 min.). Transfer the batch to a holding container to keep warm for now.

5. Heat the same pan (medium temp) to warm the rest of the oil.

6. Mince and toss in the garlic to sauté for one to two minutes. Mix in the milk and salt and wait for it to boil, continually stirring.

7. Transfer the pan to a cool burner and fold in cheese until melted. Whisk in the sour cream.

8. Combine the mixture with the fettuccine and add the shrimp and crab.

9. Warm and stir in the basil to serve.

Nutrition: Calories: 538 Protein: 40 grams Fat: 16 grams Sat. Fats: 7 grams Carbohydrates: 56 grams Sugars: 9 grams Fiber: 3 grams

Chick-fil-A's Chicken Biscuit

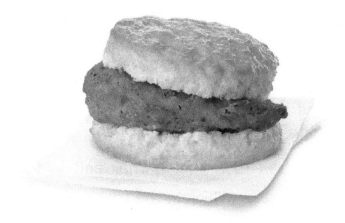

Preparation Time: 60 min

Cooking Time: 50 minutes

Servings: 4

Ingredients:

The Biscuits:

- A-P flour (1.25 cups)
- Salt (.5 tsp.)
- Baking powder (1 tbsp.)
- Chilled unsalted butter (.25 cup)
- Cold buttermilk (.5 cup)
- Honey (.5 tbsp.)
- The Chicken:
- Dill pickle juice (.33 cup)

- Milk (2/3 cup)
- Boneless chicken breast (1 lb.)
- Eggs (2)
- Breadcrumbs (.75 cup)
- Powdered sugar (2 tbsp.)
- All-Pur. flour (.75 cup)
- Kosher salt (2 tsp.)
- Chili powder (.25 tsp.)
- Black pepper (.5 tsp.)
- Peanut oil

Directions:

1. Prepare the Biscuits: Preheat the oven at 425° Fahrenheit.
2. Measure and add the salt, flour, and baking powder in a food processor, pulsing to mix.
3. Cube and add the butter to create coarse crumbs, dumping it into a mixing container. Scoop a hole in the center to add the honey and buttermilk. Do not overwork it, stirring with a spatula until just combined.
4. Lightly flour a cutting board. Scoop the dough onto the board, rolling it until it is about one inch thick. Knead the dough to process six times.

5. Gently roll the dough into a rectangular shape until it's about 1/2-inch thick.

6. Use a three-inch biscuit cutter to make eight biscuits. Scoop the scraps to make another biscuit.

7. Add a layer of parchment baking paper over a baking sheet. Gently brush each biscuit with buttermilk. Set a timer to bake until the tops are golden (15 min.). Transfer to the top of the stovetop and brush with melted butter.

8. Prepare the Chicken: Pound the chicken breasts into a 1/2-inch thickness and cut in half. Put them into a zipper-type bag with the whisked eggs, milk, and pickle juice. Marinate the chicken in the fridge for about half an hour.

9. Toss the breadcrumbs into the food processor and pulse until they're finely crushed. Toss and whisk the salt, flour, breadcrumbs, sugar, black pepper, and chili powder in a mixing bowl.

10. Dip the breasts of chicken in the mixture and wait for about five minutes before cooking them.

11. Add oil to a cast-iron skillet (1/2-inch deep) using the medium temperature setting.

Cook the chicken in batches if needed for about two to three minutes per side.

12.   Slice the freshly made biscuit and serve promptly.

Nutrition: Calories: 552 Protein: 34 grams Fat: 20 grams Sat. Fats: 10 grams Carbohydrates: 58 grams Sugars: 11 grams Fiber: 2 grams

Chick-fil-A's Chicken Egg & Cheese Biscuit

Preparation Time: 45-50 min

Cooking Time: 40 minutes

Servings: 5

Ingredients:

- Peanut oil for frying (6 cups)

Wet Mixture for The Chicken:

- Pickle juice (.5 cup)
- Whole milk (.5 cup)
- Garlic & onion powder (.5 tsp. each)
- Chicken thighs (2.5 lb.)
- Egg (1)

Dry Mixture for The Chicken:

- A-P flour (3 cups)
- Baking powder (2 tbsp.)
- Kosher salt (1 tbsp.)
- Powdered sugar (.25 cup)
- Paprika (1 tbsp.)
- Chili powder (2 tsp.)
- Refrigerated buttermilk biscuits (6 oz.)
- Cheesy Eggs:
- Cooking oil spray (as needed)

- Milk (.25 cup)
- Large eggs (8)
- Kosher salt (2 tsp.)
- Cheddar cheese (5 slices)

Directions:

1. Warm the oven according to directions on the package of biscuits.
2. Attach a deep-frying thermometer to the side of a large heavy-bottomed pot or Dutch oven. Warm about 2.5 inches of oil using the medium temperature setting (325° Fahrenheit). Cover a baking tray using a few paper towels.
3. Whisk the wet fixings in a medium bowl. Place the chicken into marinade.
4. As the oil heats, whisk the dry ingredients.
5. Reserving the marinade, transfer the chicken to a bowl.
6. Whisk the egg into the marinade. Dip the chicken into the egg mixture, one piece at a time, shaking off excess egg mixture. Dredge chicken pieces in the flour mix, making sure to coat evenly on both sides.
7. Repeat the breading process (egg mixture to flour mixture) one more time, and set chicken aside.

---

8. Once the oil is heated, cook the chicken for about two to three minutes on each side until well done.

9. As the chicken cooks, prepare the biscuits according to package directions. Place cooked chicken on the prepared baking sheet to drain. Set biscuits aside.

10. Scramble the Eggs: Reset the oven temperature at 350° Fahrenheit. Generously spray a small rimmed baking sheet (9x13) with cooking oil spray. In a medium bowl, reserving the sliced cheddar cheese, whisk the folded egg fixings until pale in color and frothy.

11. Dump the egg mixture into the baking sheet. Cook until the mixture is slightly wobbly, but set in the center, about six to eight minutes, rotating the pan halfway through.

12. Cover the baking tray with a cutting board for about four minutes, or until the egg is set in center, but still tender.

13. With two hands, use kitchen towels to the sandwich baking sheet and cutting board. Flip the "sandwich" over, placing the board on the kitchen counter.

14. Lift the pan and slice the cooked egg crosswise into five even strips. Gently fold each slice in half lengthwise and transfer, using a thin spatula, back onto the baking tray. Top with cheese to bake for two to three minutes, or until the cheese is melted.

15. Split each biscuit in half and top each with chicken, egg, and remaining biscuit top. Serve immediately.

Nutrition: Calories: 3171.5 Protein: 46.1 grams Fat: 2684 grams Sat. Fats: 58.6 grams Carbohydrates: 83.7 grams Sugars: 10.6 grams Fiber: 3.2 grams

Chick-fil-A's Sandwich

Preparation Time: 55 min

Cooking Time: 40 minutes

Servings: 4

Ingredients:

- Hamburger buns (4split)
- Lettuce (1 head)
- Dill pickle (20 slices)
- Sliced tomato (1)
- Chicken breasts (2)
- Milk divided (1.5 cups)
- Dill pickle juice (1 cup)
- Egg (1 large)
- All-purpose flour (.5 cup)
- Kosher salt and freshly cracked black pepper (as desired)
- Confectioners' sugar (1 tbsp.)
- Peanut oil (1 cup)

Directions:

1. Slice the breast of chicken in half horizontally on a cutting board, trimming away the fat.
2. Whisk the pickle juice and 1/2 cup milk. Toss in the chicken and marinate it for about 30 minutes. Drain well.

3. Prepare a skillet using the medium-temperature setting to warm the oil.

4. Prepare another container and whisk egg and last cup of milk. Fold in the chicken to coat.

5. In a gallon-sized zipper-type bag, combine the flour, salt, pepper, and confectioners' sugar. Toss in the chicken and shake to cover.

6. Arrange the chicken in the skillet and fry for four to five minutes. (Prepare in batches if needed and drain on paper towels.)

7. Serve the chicken promptly on buns with lettuce, pickles, and tomatoes.

Nutrition: Calories: 454.6 Carbohydrates: 44.2 grams Protein: 28.6 grams Fat: 18.2 grams Sat. Fats: 2.9 grams Sugars: 7.6 grams Fiber: 5.1 grams

Chick-fil-A's Market Salad

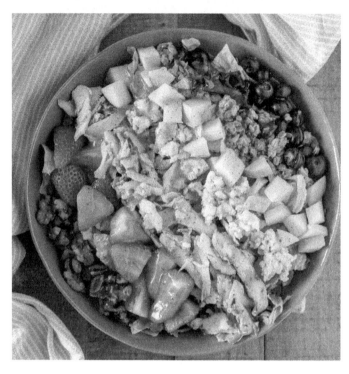

Preparation

Time: 25 min

Cooking Time: 10 minutes

Servings: 4

Ingredients:

- Chicken breast (2)
- Olive oil (1 tbsp.)
- Coarse black pepper (1/8 tsp.)
- Kosher salt (.25 tsp.)
- Paprika (.25 tsp.)
- Cayenne pepper (1/8 tsp.)

- Chopped spring salad mix (16 cups)
- Blueberries (1 cup)
- Chopped Granny Smith apple (1)
- Strawberries (1 cup halved)
- Crumbled blue cheese (.5 cup)
- Granola (1 cup)
- Roasted walnuts (1 cup)
- Zesty apple cider vinaigrette (1 cup below)
- Olive oil (.66 cup)
- Lime juice (3 tbsp.)
- Honey (.25 cup)
- Apple cider vinegar (.25 cup)
- Black pepper (.5 tsp.)
- Garlic powder (.5 tsp.)
- Salt (1 tsp.)

Directions:

1. Combine the oil, chicken, cayenne, black pepper, salt, and pepper.
2. Warm a skillet using the medium temperature setting. Cook the chicken for five to eight minutes per side. Cool the chicken and prepare the salad.
3. Prepare the vinaigrette using the listed fixings and shake it thoroughly before using it.

4. Layer the lettuce, cabbage, carrots, strawberries, blueberries, apple, walnuts, granola, and blue cheese. Thinly slice and add the chicken.

5. Spritz with the chilled dressing and serve.

Nutrition: Calories: 311 Protein: 30 grams Fat: 12 grams Sat. Fats: 4 grams Carbohydrates: 22 grams Sugars: 13 grams Fiber: 5 grams

Chick-fil-A's Sweet Carrot Salad

Preparation Time: 40 min

Cooking Time: 0 minutes

Servings: 8

Ingredients:

- Grated carrots (1 lb.)
- Raisins (.5 cup)
- Crushed pineapple (1 cup)
- Lemon juice (1 dash)
- Honey (1 tbsp.)
- Mayonnaise (2 tbsp.)

Directions:

1. Chop/mince the carrots, pineapple, and raisins.
2. Mix in the honey, lemon juice, and mayo.
3. Pop it in the fridge for at least half an hour before serving.

Nutrition: Calories: 105 Protein: 1 gram Fat: 2.9 grams Sat. Fats: 0.4 grams Carbohydrates: 20.6 grams Sugars: 15.3 grams Fiber: 2.2 grams

Chick-fil-A's Chick Nuggets

Preparation Time: 45 min

Cooking Time: 25 minutes

Servings: 4

Ingredients:

- Large eggs (2)
- Milk (1 cup)
- Chicken breast (1-inch cubes1 lb.)
- Flour (.75 cup)
- Breadcrumbs (.75 cup)
- Powdered sugar (2 tbsp.)
- White pepper (.5 tsp.)
- Kosher salt (2 tsp.)
- Chili powder (.25 tsp.)
- Peanut oil (3-inches in the skillet)

Directions:

1. Toss the breadcrumbs into a food processor, pulsing until they're fine.
2. Use a zipper-type baggie and add the pieces of chicken, whisked, eggs, and milk.
3. Place the marinated chicken in the fridge for about 15-20 minutes.
4. Pour three inches of oil into a Dutch oven and heat using the med-high temperature setting.

5. Measure and whisk the powdered sugar, flour, breadcrumbs, salt, white pepper, and chili powder into a shallow dish.

6. Dip the chicken into the flour mix. Wait a minute and fry in batches (2-3 min.). Transfer them onto a baking tray to serve promptly. Don't use towels to drain because it could soften/steam the nuggets.

Nutrition: Calories: 379 Protein: 33 grams Fat: 8 grams Sat. Fats: 2 grams Carbohydrates: 39 grams Sugars: 8 grams Fiber: 1 gram

Chick-fil-A's Honey Mustard Grilled Chicken

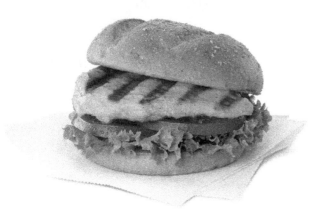

Preparation Time: 35 min

Cooking Time: 20 minutes

Servings: 4

Ingredients:

- Dijon mustard (.33 cup)
- Honey (.25 cup)
- Mayonnaise (2 tbsp.)
- Steak sauce (1 tsp.)
- Chicken breast halves (4no skin or bones)

Directions:

1. Lightly oil the grate and warm the grill using the medium temperature setting.
2. Prepare a shallow dish with the steak sauce, mayo, honey, and mustard. Set aside a portion for basting and rest for the coating sauce.
3. Grill the chicken for about 20 minutes, turning intermittently.
4. Baste using the reserved sauce the last ten minutes of the cooking cycle.

Nutrition: Calories: 265.9 Protein: 24.7 grams Fat: 8.3 grams Sat. Fats: 1.6 grams Carbohydrates: 22 grams Sugars: 17.5 grams Fiber: 0.1 grams

SOUPS AND STEWS RECIPES

Ruby Tuesday® White Chicken Chili

Preparation Time: 10 minutes

Cooking Time: 2 hours

Servings: 8

Ingredients:

- 1-pound great northern beans
- 6 cups chicken stock
- 2 medium chopped onions
- 2 minced garlic cloves
- 6 cups diced cooked chicken
- 1 cup salsa
- 2 seeded and diced jalapeño peppers
- 2 diced chili peppers
- 1 1/2 teaspoons oregano
- 2 teaspoons cumin
- 1/4 teaspoon cayenne pepper

- 1 tablespoon vegetable oil
- Salt, to taste

Directions:

1. Soak beans in water overnight. Drain the beans the next day. In a large stock pot, add the chicken stock, beans and half the onions and garlic.
2. Simmer for 2 hours until the beans become soft, stir it frequently. Add the salsa and chicken.
3. Sauté spices, peppers and the remaining garlic and onions in oil for 3-4 minutes in a large skillet. Add the chili, salt and pepper to the pot. Simmer it for 1 more hour.

Nutrition: Calories 224; Fat 5g; Carbs 25g; Protein 18g

T.G.I. Friday® Broccoli Cheese Soup

Preparation Time: 5 minutes

Cooking Time: 30 minutes

Servings: 6

Ingredients:

- 4 cups chicken broth
- 1 cup half-and-half
- 1 cup water
- 4 slices American cheese
- 1/2 cup flour
- 1/2 teaspoon dried onion flakes
- 1/4 teaspoon black pepper
- 4 1/2 cups bite-size broccoli florets

Directions:

1. Combine all the ingredients except the broccoli into a large soup pot. Bring to a boil, stirring constantly. Reduce to a simmer. Add the broccoli and simmer for 15 minutes, or until the broccoli is tender. Garnish with shredded Cheddar cheese.

Nutrition: Calories 587; Fat 25g; Carbs 19g; Protein 9g

T.G.I. Friday® French Onion Soup

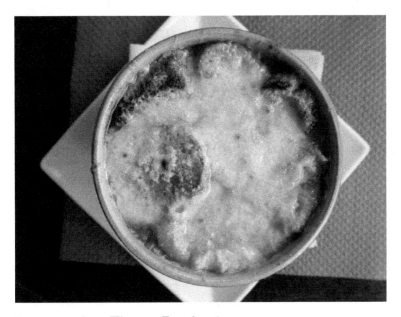

Preparation Time: 5 minutes

Cooking Time: 35 minutes

Servings: 4

Ingredients:

- 2 tablespoons butter
- 4 medium sliced onions
- 4 cups beef broth
- 1 tablespoon Worcestershire sauce
- 1/4 teaspoon black pepper
- Dash of dried thyme
- 1 cup French bread cubes
- 1/2 cup shredded mozzarella cheese

Directions:

1. Melt butter in a 2-quart saucepan. Add the onions and cook 20 minutes, stirring occasionally. Add the broth, Worcestershire sauce, pepper, and thyme. Increase the heat to medium-high and bring to a boil. Reduce the heat to low, cover, and simmer for 5 minutes. Divide soup into 4 individual serving crocks. Place the bread cubes on top of the soup and then add the cheese. Put the soup bowls under the broiler to melt the cheese until it turns slightly brown.

Nutrition: Calories 310; Fat 27g; Carbs 14g; Protein 6g

PF Chang® Spicy Chicken Noodle Soup

Preparation Time: 15 minutes

Cooking Time: 15 minutes

Servings: 4-6

Ingredients:

- 2 quarts chicken stock
- 1 tablespoon granulated sugar
- 3 tablespoons white vinegar
- 2 cloves garlic, minced
- 1 tablespoon ginger, freshly minced
- 1/4 cup of soy sauce
- Sriracha sauce to taste
- Red pepper flakes to taste
- 1 lbs. Boneless chicken breast, cut into thin 2–3-inch pieces
- 3 tablespoons cornstarch
- Salt to taste
- 1 cup mushrooms, sliced
- 1 cup grape tomatoes, halved
- 3 green onions, sliced
- 2 tablespoons fresh cilantro, chopped

- 1/2-pound pasta, cooked to just under package directions and drained

Directions:

1. Add the chicken stock, sugar, vinegar, garlic, ginger, soy sauce, Sriracha and red pepper flakes to a large saucepan. Boil it and then lower the heat to a simmer. Let cook for 5 minutes.

2. Season chicken with salt to taste. In a resalable bag, combine the chicken and the cornstarch. Shake to coat. Add the chicken to the simmering broth a piece at a time. Then add the mushrooms. Continue to cook for another 5 minutes.

3. Stir in the tomatoes, green onions, cilantro, and cooked pasta. Serve with additional cilantro.

Nutrition: Calories 500; Protein 32g; Fat 8g; Carbohydrate: 73g

Panera Broccoli Cheddar Soup

Preparation Time: 15 minutes

Cooking Time: 50 minutes

Servings: 8

Ingredients:

- 1 tablespoon butter
- 1/2 onion, diced
- 1/4 cup melted butter
- 1/4 cup flour
- 2 cups of milk
- 2 cups chicken stock
- 1 1/2 cup broccoli florets, diced
- 1 cup carrots, cut into thin strips
- 1 stalk celery, sliced
- 2 1/2 cups Cheddar cheese, grated
- Salt and pepper, to taste

Directions:

1. Melt tablespoon of butter in a frying pan and cook onion over medium heat for 5 minutes or until caramelized. Set aside. In a saucepan, mix melted butter and flour, then cook on medium-low heat. Add 1 or 2 tablespoons milk to the flour to prevent from burning—Cook for at least 3 minutes or until smooth.

2. Gently pour the rest of the milk in with the flour while stirring. Mix in chicken stock. Simmer for 20 minutes or until thick and well blended. Toss in the broccoli, carrots, cooked onion, and celery. Cook for an additional 20 minutes or until vegetables turns soft. Mix in cheese and stir until the cheese is completely melted—season with salt and pepper, to taste. Transfer into individual bowls. Serve.

Nutrition: Calories 304; Fat 23g; Carbs 11g; Protein 14g

Outback® Walkabout Soup

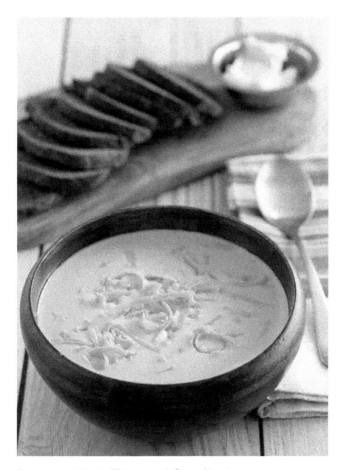

Preparation Time: 10 minutes

Cooking Time: 45 minutes

Servings: 4

Ingredients:

- Thick white Sauce
- 3 tablespoons butter
- 3 tablespoons flour

- 1/4 teaspoon salt
- 1 1/2 cups whole milk
- Soup
- 2 cups yellow sweet onions, thinly sliced
- 3 tablespoons butter
- 1 can (14.5 ounces) chicken broth
- 1/2 teaspoon salt
- 1/4 teaspoon fresh ground black pepper
- 2 chicken bouillon cubes
- 1/4 cup Velveeta cubes, diced, packed
- 1 1/2-1¾ cups white sauce (recipe above)
- Cheddar cheese for garnish, shredded
- Crusty bread for serving

Directions:

1. Make the thick white sauce first. Make a roux by cooking melted butter and flour over medium heat. Slowly pour the milk onto the roux, a little at a time, while constantly stirring the mixture. When the mixture reaches a pudding-like consistency, remove it from heat and set aside. In a soup pot, sauté the onions in the butter over medium heat until they become translucent.

2. Add the rest of the ingredients, except the cheese and white sauce, to the pot and mix

everything together. When the mixture has heated up completely, add the cheese and white sauce. Bring the entire mixture to a simmer on medium-low heat. Continuously stir the soup until everything is completely mixed together.

3. When the cheese has melted, turn the heat lower and continue to cook the soup for another 30 to 45 minutes. Ladle the soup into bowls and garnish with cheese. Serve with a side of bread.

Nutrition: Calories 329, Fat 25 g, Carbs 17g, Protein 6 g

Chevy® Chipotle Slaw

Preparation Time: 10 minutes

Cooking Time: 0 minutes

Servings: 6

Ingredients:

- 3 cups finely shredded white cabbage
- 3 cups finely shredded red cabbage
- ¾ cup Sweet Chipotle Dressing
- Sweet Chipotle Dressing
- 1 tablespoon diced onion
- 2 teaspoons minced garlic
- 1 chipotle pepper in adobo sauce, diced
- 1 tablespoon adobo sauce
- 2 tablespoons mustard
- 1/2 teaspoon ground cumin
- 1/2 cup diced fresh tomatoes
- 2 tablespoons chopped cilantro
- 2/3Cup of seasoned rice wine vinegar
- 1/4 teaspoon black pepper
- 1 teaspoon salt
- 2 tablespoons honey
- 1/2 cup olive oil

Directions:

1. Shred the cabbage. Put it in a large bowl. Combine all the dressing ingredients EXCEPT the oil until smooth in a blender or food processor.
2. While the blender is running, drizzle in the oil to make an emulsion.
3. Pour ¾ cup of the dressing over the cabbage and toss to coat.
4. Put the remaining dressing in an airtight container and store it in the fridge for up to 1 week.

Nutrition: Calories 100; Protein 1g; Fat 10g; Carbs 6g

Café Rio® Black Beans

Preparation Time: 10 minutes

Cooking Time: 30 minutes

Servings: 8

Ingredients:

- 2 tablespoons olive oil
- 3 cloves garlic, minced
- 1 jalapeño pepper, minced
- 2 (15-ounce) cans black beans (one can drain, one with liquid)
- 2 teaspoons cumin
- 12 ounces tomato juice
- 1 teaspoon salt
- 1/2 teaspoon black pepper
- 1/4 cup chopped cilantro

Directions:

1. In a large non-stick skillet over medium heat, warm the oil and sauté the garlic and jalapeño until fragrant. Add the beans and cumin. Bring the mixture to a simmer for 5-10 minutes, until some of the liquid has evaporated. Stir in the tomato juice, salt, pepper, and cilantro. Cook to heat through, and serve.

Nutrition: Calories 153; Protein 9g; Fat 3g; Carbs 25g

Applebee® Cheese Chicken Tortilla Soup

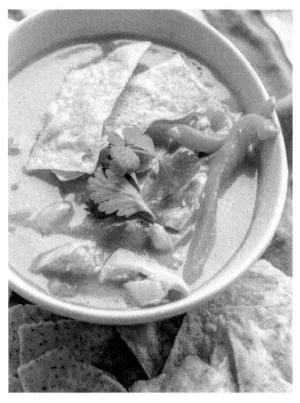

Preparation Time: 10 minutes

Cooking Time: 40 minutes

Servings: 6-8

Ingredients:

- 2 tablespoons vegetable oil
- 2 teaspoons minced garlic
- 1 medium chopped onion
- 1/4 cup chopped green pepper

- 1 (15 ounces) can tomato purée
- 4 cups chicken stock
- 1 teaspoon sugar
- 1/2 teaspoon salt
- 1 teaspoon chili powder
- 1 teaspoon Worcestershire sauce
- 10 (6") yellow corn tortillas
- 4 tablespoons flour
- 1/2 cup of water
- 1-pound cooked chicken
- 1 cup cream
- 1/4 cup nonfat sour cream
- 8 ounces Velveeta cheese, cut into 1" cubes

Directions:

1. Add oil and sauté garlic, onions, and green peppers in a large stockpot over medium heat. Add chicken stock, tomato purée, sugar, salt, chili powder, and Worcestershire sauce to the pot.
2. Bring to a boil, reduce the heat and simmer for 20 minutes. Cut tortillas into 1/4" strips and bake in the oven at 400°F for 6-8 minutes until crispy.

3. In a small bowl, mix flour and water, then whisk into the soup. Add chicken and cream, bring to a boil, and then simmer for 5 minutes. Put it into bowls and garnish with the cheese, sour cream, and tortilla strips.

Nutrition: Calories 190 Protein 9g; Fat 9g; Carbs 18g

California Pizza Kitchen® Pea and Barley Soup

Preparation Time: 10 minutes

Cooking Time: 2 hours and 20 minutes

Servings: 8

Ingredients:

- 2 cups split peas
- 6 cups of water
- 4 cups chicken broth
- 1/3 cup minced onion
- 1 large clove minced garlic
- 2 teaspoons lemon juice
- 1 teaspoon salt
- 1 teaspoon granulated sugar
- 1/4 teaspoon dried parsley
- 1/4 teaspoon white pepper
- Dash dried thyme
- 1/2 cup barley
- 6 cups of water
- 2 medium diced carrots
- 1/2 stalk diced celery

Directions:

1. Rinse and drain the split peas and add them to a large pot with 6 cups of water, chicken broth, onion, garlic, lemon juice, salt, sugar, parsley, pepper, and thyme. Bring to a boil. Reduce heat and simmer for 75 minutes, or until the peas becomes soft.

2. Combine the barley with 6 cups of water in a saucepan while the peas are cooking. Bring to a boil, reduce heat, and simmer for 75 minutes, or until the barley is soft and most of the water has been absorbed.

3. Drain the barley in a colander and add it to the split peas. Add the celery and carrots and continue to simmer the soup for 15-30 minutes, or until the carrots are tender. Stir occasionally. Turn off the heat, cover the soup, and let it sit for 10-15 minutes before serving.

Nutrition: Calories 340; Protein 66g; Fat 23g; Carbs 3g

SNACK RECIPES

Great American Cookies Snickerdoodles

Preparation Time: 25 Minutes

Cooking Time: 14 Minutes

Servings: 6

Ingredients:

- 1 cup Crisco shortening, butter flavor
- 1 cup white sugar
- 2/3 cup brown sugar, packed
- 2–3 organic eggs
- 1 tablespoon vanilla
- 3½ cups flour
- ¼ teaspoon salt
- 1 teaspoon baking soda
- ¾ teaspoon cream of tartar
  Topping Ingredients
- ¼ cup white sugar
- ½ teaspoon cinnamon

Directions:

1. Preheat oven to 320°F.
2. Combine cream of tartar, both sugars, and shortening together in a bowl and blend with a hand beater.
3. Add eggs, vanilla, salt, flour, and baking soda.
4. Mix all ingredients well.
5. Rest the dough for 3 hours in the fridge.
6. In a small bowl, add topping ingredients and mix well.
7. Roll the dough by hand and make small golf-ball-shaped rounds.
8. Roll the balls in the topping ingredients.
9. Once they're coated, place them on a parchment-lined baking sheet.
10. Press the balls to flatten slightly.
11. Bake for 10–14 minutes.
12. Serve once cooled.

Nutrition: Calories 689, Total fat 18.2 g, Carbs 122.2 g, Protein 9.4 g,

Sodium 335 mg

Little Debbie Star Crunch

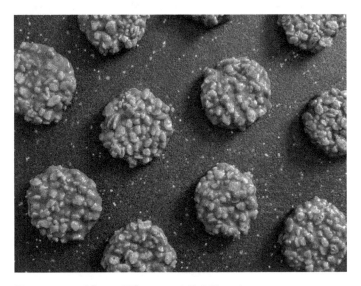

Preparation Time: 15 Minutes

Cooking Time: 3 to 4 Minutes

Servings: 6

Ingredients:

- 11 ounces caramel bits
- 1/3 cup butter, unsalted
- 3 cups marshmallows
- 2 cups Rice Krispies cereal
- 2 cups milk chocolate chips, melted
- ¼ cup vegetable shortening

Directions:

1. Line a baking sheet with parchment paper.

2. Melt caramel bites in the microwave for 1 minute, stir, and then add butter and microwave for 1 more minute.
3. Add marshmallows and melt in the microwave for about 1-2 minutes.
4. While still hot, add the cereal and stir the mixture well.
5. Make small discs of batter by hand.
6. Place the discs on a baking sheet then cover with plastic wrap.
7. Cool for 2 hours in the refrigerator until firm.
8. Melt shortening then chocolate chips in the microwave for 1 minutes, stir and continue heating until smooth.
9. Dip the discs in chocolate until coated well.
10. Cool in the fridge for 2 hours, until hard.
11. Serve.

Nutrition: Calories 150, Total fat 6 g, Carbs 22 g, Protein 1 g, Sodium 65 mg

Oreo Cookies

Preparation Time: 40 Minutes

Cooking Time: 30 Minutes

Servings: 8

Ingredients:

Ingredients for Dough

- 1½ cups cocoa powder
- 1 1/3 cups all-purpose flour,
- 2 tablespoons butter, softened
- 1½ cups granulated sugar
- 3 large eggs
- 1 teaspoon vanilla extract

Ingredients for Filling

- 1 tablespoon butter, softened
- 1/3 cup vegetable shortening
- 2 cups sugar
- 2 teaspoons vanilla extract

Directions:

1. Mix the dough ingredients with a hand beater to make the dough.
2. Divide the dough into two pieces and place one piece between two sheets of parchment paper.
3. Roll the dough into a ¼-inch-thick rectangle.
4. Repeat with the other piece of dough.

---

5. Chill in the fridge for a limited hour.

6. Cut the prepared dough into small circles.

7. Preheat oven to 340°F.

8. Place all the circles on a greased baking sheet.

9. Bake for 20 minutes.

10.   Meanwhile, mix all the filling ingredients.

11.   Take away the cookies from the oven and allow to cool.

12.   Top the cookies with the filling mixture and then place and press another cookie on top to make an Oreo cookie.

13.   Repeat with all cookies.

Nutrition: Calories 850, Total fat 47 g, Carbs 112 g, Protein 7.8 g, Sodium 278 mg

Nabisco SnackWells Banana Snack Bars

Preparation Time: 35 Minutes

Cooking Time: 25 Minutes

Servings: 20

Ingredients:

- 2 egg whites
- 1 cup + 5 tablespoons sugar
- 2 tablespoons dark brown sugar
- 2 tablespoons molasses
- 1½ cups banana puree
- 3 tablespoons shortening
- ¼ cup whole milk
- ½ teaspoon vanilla butternut extract
- 1½ cups all-purpose flour
- ½ teaspoon salt
- ¼ teaspoon baking soda

Directions:

1. Preheat oven to 375°F.
2. Take a large bowl and whisk eggs with a hand beater until fluffy.
3. Add the remaining ingredients one by one and mix until a smooth textured mixture is obtained.

4. Lightly grease a 9×12-inch pan with oil.

5. Dump the mixture into the pan.

6. Sprinkle with a light coating of sugar.

7. Bake for 25 minutes.

8. Once brown, take it out.

9. Let cool.

10.   Cut into 20 snack bars and enjoy.

Nutrition: Calories 101, Total fat 2.2, Carbs 19.4 g, Protein 1.7 g,

Sodium 80 mg

Girl Scout Samoa Cookies

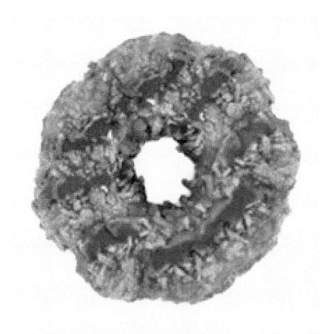

Preparation Time: 15-20 Minutes

Cooking Time: 5 Minutes

Servings: 10

Ingredients:

- 24 shortbread cookies
- ¼ cup butter
- 1/3 cup sugar
- ½ cup corn syrup
- 1 teaspoon vanilla extract
- ½ cup condensed milk
- 4 cups coconut flakes

- ½ cup chocolate chips, melted

Directions:

1. Add sugar, butter, and corn syrup in a saucepan.
2. Heat the saucepan and cook for 3 minutes.
3. Slowly add the condensed milk.
4. Mix and remove from heat.
5. Add the vanilla.
6. Mix well until creamy.
7. Add coconut flakes
8. Spoon the mixture over shortbread cookies.
9. Let cool.
10. Place in refrigerator to cool some more.
11. Dip the cookies in the melted chocolate chips.
12. Place on flat paper.
13. Let harden, then serve.

Nutrition: Calories 630, Total fat 31 g, Carbs 87 g, Protein 7.8 g, Sodium 402 mg

Lemon Cooler Cookies

Preparation Time: 40 Minutes

Cooking Time: 25 Minutes

Servings: 6

Ingredients:

Main Ingredients

- 1/3 cup powdered sugar
- 1/3 cup sugar
- ½ cup shortening
- 1–2 large eggs
- 1 teaspoon vanilla
- ¼ teaspoon salt
- 1 1/3 cups cake flour
- 1 1/3 teaspoons baking powder
- 2 tablespoons water

Sugar Powder Ingredients

- 1 cup powdered sugar
- 1/3 teaspoon Kool-Aid lemonade mix, unsweetened

Directions:

1. Preheat oven to 325°F.
2. Take a bowl and mix all the main ingredients.
3. Form a dough, roll it into approximately ¾-inch balls, and then flatten the balls a bit.

4. Place balls on a greased pan.

5. Bake for 25 minutes.

6. Combine all the powder ingredients in a Ziploc bag.

7. Remove cookies from the oven and then put in the Ziploc bag.

8. Shake to coat the cookies.

9. Serve and enjoy.

Nutrition: Calories 460, Total fat 18.2 g, Carbs 73, Protein 3.8 g, Sodium 80 mg

Pepperidge Farm Soft Baked Snickerdoodles

Preparation Time: 25 Minutes

Cooking Time: 14 Minutes

Servings: 6

Ingredients:

- 1/3 cup butter, melted
- 1 cup dark brown sugar
- 2 large eggs
- 2 teaspoons vanilla extract
- 1 cup all-purpose flour
- ½ teaspoon baking soda
- ½ teaspoon cream of tartar
- 1/3 teaspoon salt
  Topping Ingredients
- 2 tablespoons white sugar
- 2 teaspoons ground cinnamon

Directions:

1. Combine topping ingredients in a bowl.
2. Preheat the oven to 320°F.
3. Combine butter, brown sugar, eggs, and vanilla in a bowl and blend with a beater.

4. In a separate bowl, add flour, cream of tartar, salt and baking soda.

5. Combine ingredients from both bowls to make a smooth dough.

6. Measure 1 tablespoon of dough then roll into a small ball.

7. Make the small balls of all the dough and then press the balls into the cinnamon-and-sugar mixture.

8. Place the balls on a baking sheet then bake for 20 minutes. Don't overcook.

9. Take out the cookies and let cool.

10.   Serve.

Nutrition: Calories 304, Total fat 12 g, Carbs 44 g, Protein 4.4 g,

Sodium 325 mg

Reese's Peanut Butter Cups

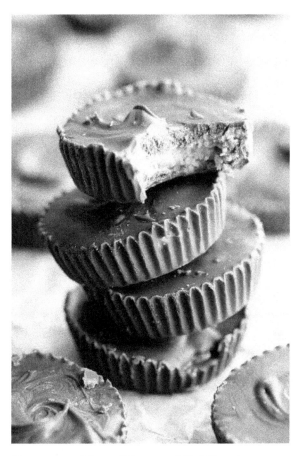

Preparation Time: 15 Minutes

Cooking Time: 2 Minutes

Servings: 10

Ingredients:

- Salt, pinch
- 1½ cups peanut butter
- 1 cup confectioners' sugar
- 20 ounces milk chocolate chips

Directions:

1. Take a medium bowl and mix the salt, peanut butter, and sugar until firm.
2. Place the chocolate chips in a microwave-safe bowl and microwave for 2 minutes to melt.
3. Grease the muffin tin with oil spray and spoon some of the melted chocolate into each muffin cup.
4. Take a spoon and draw the chocolate up to the edges of the muffin cups until all sides are coated.
5. Cool in the refrigerator for few hours.
6. Once chocolate is solid, spread about 1 teaspoon of peanut butter onto each cup.
7. Leave space to fill the edges of the cups.
8. Create the final layer by pouring melted chocolate on top of each muffin cup.
9. Let sit at room temperature until cool.
10. Refrigerate for a few hours until firm.
11. Take away the cups from the muffin tray and serve.

Nutrition: Calories 455, Total fat 21.7 g, Carbs 59 g, Protein 9.7 g,
Sodium 384 mg

Nestlé Baby Ruth Candy Bar

Preparation Time: 25 Minutes

Cooking Time: 12 Minutes

Servings: 10

Ingredients:

- ½ cup whole milk
- 10 unwrapped caramels
- 2 tablespoons light corn syrup
- 2 teaspoons butter
- ½ teaspoon vanilla extract
- ¼ teaspoon salt
- 1½ cups powdered sugar
  Other Ingredients
- 40 unwrapped caramels
- 2 teaspoons water
- 4 cups peanuts, dry roasted
- 20 ounces chocolate chips

Directions:

1. Combine all the main fixings excluding for the powdered sugar in a saucepan and heat on low heat.
2. Stir to combine all the ingredients well.
3. Add half of the powdered sugar and reserve the rest.

4. Heat for a few minutes.

5. Turn off the heat.

6. Add the remaining sugar and mix it in with a spoon.

7. Once thickened, take a small portion and form it into a roll using your hands.

8. Repeat with the remaining mixture.

9. Place all rolls on wax paper.

10. Combine caramels with water in a pan and heat.

11. Once caramels melt, turn off the heat.

12. Pour peanuts onto a baking sheet.

13. Coat the rolls with a fine layering of caramel on every side.

14. Quickly set the caramel-coated roll down onto the layered peanuts.

15. Roll it to stick the peanuts to the surface of the candy. The peanuts should cover all sides of the roll.

16. Place the peanut-coated candy onto wax paper.

17. Repeat with all the rolls.

18. Place in the refrigerator for 1 hour.

19. Microwave the chocolate chips for 2 minutes to melt.

20.   Drop a refrigerated candy bar into the melted milk chocolate.

21.   Cover it on all sides and then place on wax paper.

22.   Repeat with all bars.

23.   Let sit until solid.

24.   Serve and enjoy.

Nutrition: Calories 1680, Total fat 86 g, Carbs 199 g, Protein 29 g,

Sodium 349 mg

DESSERT RECIPES

Starbucks Caramel Frappuccino Copycat

Preparation Time: 4 minutes

Cooking Time: 13 minutes

Serving: 1

Ingredients

- 1 cup strong brewed coffee, cooled
- 1 cup 1% milk
- 1 cup of ice cubes
- 1 Teaspoon sugar free caramel syrup
- ¼ cup low-fat vanilla frozen yogurt
- ½ Teaspoon agave syrup

Direction

1. Blend all the ingredients in a blender on high until creamy.

Nutrition 175 calories 17g Fat 9g Protein

Copycat Zaxby's Brownie

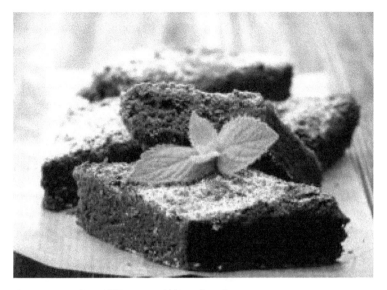

Preparation Time: 14 minutes

Cooking Time: 27 minutes

Serving: 6

Ingredients

- 1/2 cup (1stick) butter
- Three eggs
- Two oz semi-sweet dark chocolate, chopped
- 1/2 cup unsweetened cocoa powder
- 1 1/2 teaspoon vanilla
- 3/4 cup sugar
- 1/2 cup all-purpose flour
- 3/4 teaspoon salt
- 1/2 cup chopped walnuts (optional)

- One teaspoon baking powder

Direction

1. Preheat to 350 ° F on the oven.
2. Melt butter and chocolate in a saucepan set at low heat.
3. Remove from heat and whisk in the sugar, cocoa, and vanilla.
4. Attach the eggs, flour, baking powder, salt, and whisk to a smooth spot. If using, whisk in the walnuts.
5. Pour the batter into an 8 "x 8" baking pan coated with a small amount of non-stick spray.
6. Spread the batter out into a layer even.
7. Bake for 20 to 25 minutes, until almost clean comes out a toothpick inserted in the middle.

Nutrition 291 calories 24g fat 11g protein

Yogurt Parfait Copycat

Preparation Time: 17 minutes

Cooking Time: 0 minutes

Serving: 1

Ingredient

- 1/2 cup blueberries (frozen)
- 1/4 cup granola
- Two teaspoon sugar
- 4–5 mint leaves, sliced thinly
- One cup sliced strawberry
- One container (8 oz) low-fat plain Greek-style yogurt

Direction

1. In a bowl, combine the fruit, sugar, and mint and allow to sit for 3 to 4 minutes.
2. In a bowl or glass, spoon half of the yogurt, top with half of the fruit and granola, then repeat with the rest of the yogurt, fruit, and granola.
3. Pour any leftover juice over the top of the fruit.

Nutrition 330 calories 4g fat 9g protein

Cheesecake Factory Cheesecake Copycat Recipe

Preparation Time: 17 minutes

Cooking Time: 24 minutes

Serving: 5

Ingredients

For the cheesecake

- One cup of sugar
- One 1/2 cups water
- Three eggs
- 8 oz. sour cream
- One teaspoon vanilla extract
- Fresh berries, for topping

For the crust

- Ten graham crackers
- Five teaspoon butter, melted
- 8 oz. cream cheese, at room temperature

Direction

1. Preheat to 350 degrees on the oven.
2. Put the graham crackers in a bag, sealed plastic bag. Using a rolling pin, roll over the graham crackers until they're ground to a consistency similar to sand.

3. Mix the melted butter and the crushed graham crackers in a tub. Apply to a springform plate.

4. Prebake the crust for about ten minutes. Set it aside to cool.

5. While the crust cools down, use an electric mixer to whisk together the cream cheese and sugar.

6. When the cream cheese is used to work the sugar, add the sour cream and the vanilla extract—next add in the eggs, one at a time.

7. Stop mixing when the eggs are put into the cheesecake mixture. You don't want to overmix, or you crack the cheesecake in the oven.

8. Heat up the water over the stove in a kettle or pot, or even in the microwave until the water is hot.

9. In aluminum foil, wrap the bottom of the springform pan, then place it on a sheet pan with rimmed edges.

10. Pour the cheesecake mixture along with the crust into the springform pan.

11. Pour the hot water carefully into the sheet pan, creating a bath of water around the cheesecake.

12. Place the sheet saucepan in the oven (with the cheesecake on it).

13.   Bake for another 55 minutes. The cheesecake in the middle will be slightly wobbly, that's perfect.

14.   Slightly open the door of the oven, and allow it to cool for 1 hour.

15.   Let refrigerate the cheesecake for 3-4 hours, or overnight.

16.   Loosen the cheesecake rim from the saucepan with a spatula or knife. Springform pan open.

17.   Serve with fresh berries, chocolate sauce, whipped cream, or any other desired toppings!

Nutrition 410 calories 19g fat 6g protein

Chili's Molten Lava Cake

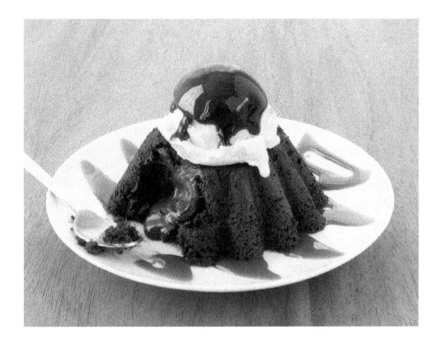

Preparation Time: 1 Hour and 25 Minutes

Cooking Time: 30 Minutes

Servings: 16

Ingredients:

- 1 14-ounce can sweeten condensed milk
- 1 12-ounce bag plus 1 cup semi-sweet chocolate chips, divided
- 4 tablespoons unsalted butter
- 1 teaspoon pure vanilla extract
- 1 pinch salt
- 1 package fudge cake mix

- 3 large eggs
- ½ cup sour cream
- 1 cup milk
- ½ cup canola oil
- Non-stick cooking spray
- 1 cup milk chocolate chips
- ¼ cup coconut oil
- Vanilla ice cream
- Caramel syrup

Directions:

1. Make hot fudge by adding condensed milk, 1 bag chocolate chips, butter, vanilla extract, and salt to a saucepan over medium heat, stirring frequently. Once boiling, continue for about 2 minutes. Turn off heat but keep stirring mixture for 1 minute more. Set aside to cool.
2. Combine cake mix, eggs, sour cream, milk, and oil in a bowl. Set aside.
3. Coat a molten cake pan or a cupcake pan with non-stick cooking spray, then pour batter into each mold. Leave about ¼ mold without batter. Bake based on package instructions. Then, invert cakes to form volcano shape then let cool.
4. Carefully cut some cake out off center of each, in a cone shape, but not all the way through.

Pour cooled hot fudge into hole. Taking the cut off cake layer, cut a thin slice on largest part then position above hot fudge like a cap.

5. As cake cools, prepare magic shells by microwaving a bowl of coconut oil and remaining chocolate chips in 30-second intervals, stirring after every interval, until melted. Wait to cool.

6. Serve cakes on a plate and top with ice cream followed by caramel, then magic shell.

Nutrition: Calories 781, Total fat 42 g, Saturated fat 22 g, Carbs 97 g,

Sugar 76 g, Fibers 1 g, Protein 8 g, Sodium 123 mg

Dunkin' Donuts Chocolate Munchkins

Preparation Time: 10 Minutes

Cooking Time: 30 Minutes

Servings: 30 munchkins

Ingredients:

- 2 tablespoons unsalted butter
- 1½ ounces unsweetened chocolate, roughly chopped
- ¼ cup buttermilk
- 1 tablespoon pure vanilla extract
- 1 large egg
- 1 cup all-purpose flour
- ¼ cup plus 2 tablespoons granulated sugar
- ¼ cup plus 2 tablespoons cocoa powder
- ¾ teaspoon baking powder
- ¼ teaspoon baking soda
- ½ teaspoon kosher salt
- Vegetable oil, for deep frying
- 2 cups powdered sugar
- 2 tablespoons milk
- 2 teaspoons pure vanilla extract

Directions:

1. To prepare dough, using a double boiler, heat butter and chocolate on top of saucepan with slightly simmering water on bottom until melted. Turning heat, then set aside to cool. Pour in buttermilk and vanilla. Mix in egg. Whisk until combined.

2. Next, mix flour, sugar, cocoa powder, baking powder, baking soda, and salt in a large bowl. Pour liquid ingredients into bowl. Stir until mixed and dough forms. Remove from bowl and wrap in plastic wrap. Keep refrigerated for 30 minutes.

3. Preheat oil to 360° F 3-inches deep in a heavy bottomed pot.

4. Scoop out small pieces out of dough and form into balls using your hands. Deep fry only a few balls at a time so as to not overcrowd pot.

5. Cook balls for about 2 to 3 minutes until cooked through. Take it from oil using a slotted spoon, then arrange onto a baking tray lined with paper towels. Let cool.

6. As munchkins cool, make glaze by combining powdered sugar, milk, and vanilla in a bowl. Whisk until it forms a smooth consistency similar to heavy cream.

7. Glaze to coat with a fork or some tongs, raising it above glaze to let drip any excess. Move to a rack over a baking tray.
8. Serve once glaze dries.

Nutrition: Calories 97, Total fat 4 g, Saturated fat 3 g, Carbs 15 g, Sugar 11 g, Fibers 1 g, Protein 1 g, Sodium 45 mg

CONCLUSION

I hope you thoroughly enjoyed each segment of Copycat Recipes Making. I also hope it was informative and provided you with all of the tools you need to achieve your goals, whatever they may be.

The next step is to decide which delicious treat you would like to prepare first. Before you proceed, you might want to consider how to store your deliciously prepared copycat recipes and be sure they are preserved until time to serve. You have several compartments in the refrigerator to keep your prepared foods. You must understand which foods store best in each location.

- Top: Don't place bread or baked products on top of the refrigerator. The heat from the fridge could cause it to spoil more quickly.
- Doors: Many refrigerators have a door to access frequently retrieved food items - available as pullout drawers without opening the main door. Non-perishable items such as

drinks, condiments, water, and other foods that don't quickly spoil could be placed here.

- Top Shelves: Once you have prepared your meals or smoothies, it is recommended to place them on the upper shelves, since these are items used most often. They also have the most consistent temperature settings.

- Lower Shelves: This is generally the coldest section of the refrigerator, making it an ideal space for dairy, eggs, and raw meat. Your unit may have individual drawers for these items to ensure a consistent temperature.

- Sealed Drawers: Fruits and veggies should get stored in this space while avoiding the mixing of meat, fruits, and vegetables. Keeping these foods together can create a risk of cross-contamination.

Other than storage, you also have the option of using your refrigerator to refrigerate food at room temperature.

When you are shopping for a new refrigerator, you should consider how many people you will be serving and how often you will need to access your foods. If it's just you, the smaller models will do fine. If you entertain guests frequently or have a big family, choosing a larger model is more practical.

If you are considering purchasing a new refrigerator, consider the following:

- A French Door or top-freezer model will allow you to refrigerate foods at room temperature. The double-door models are larger, and each door has a separate compressor for more efficient usage of space.
- The freezer section can be in the top or bottom of the unit.

Other things that you need to consider when cooking:

1. The container size is important: be sure to use a container that's big enough (not too big), as the food will expand after cooking or freezing.

2. Using a recipe box to store your copycat recipes in plastic bags is a good idea, especially if you use them frequently.

3. If the book is not in a plastic bag, you should place it in one.

4. You can also use wax paper, foil or cling wrap, but you need to be careful with the edges not to tear or rip.

5. Finally, if you have a microwave oven at home, you can use it to defrost food and cook some recipes for 15-20 minutes until the food is ready.